i

REBUILT RECOVERY
A JOURNEY WITH GOD

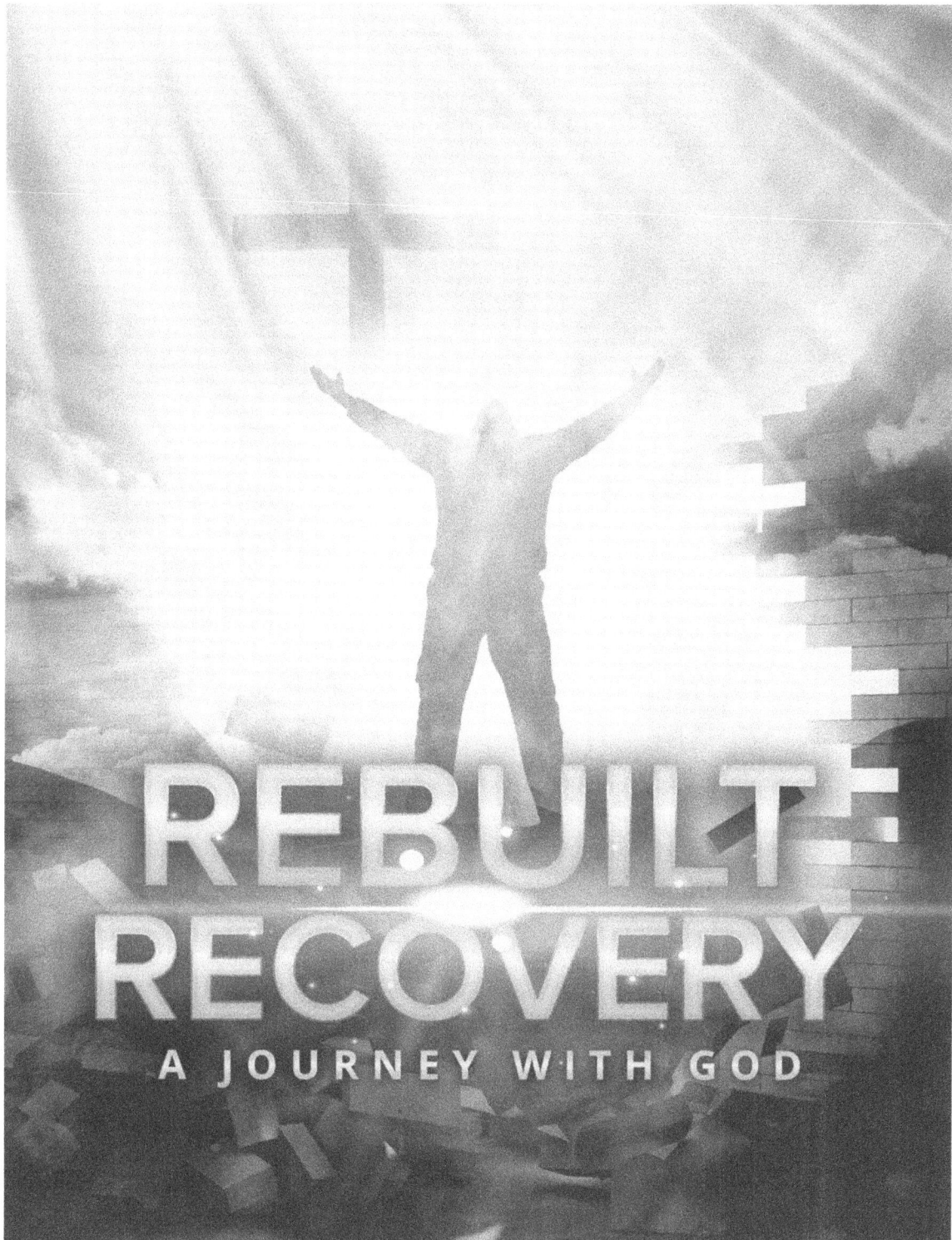

Glorious Hope Publishing

New Carlisle, Ohio

Rebuilt Recovery

A Journey with God

Book 3 – Knowing God

By: Heather L. Phipps

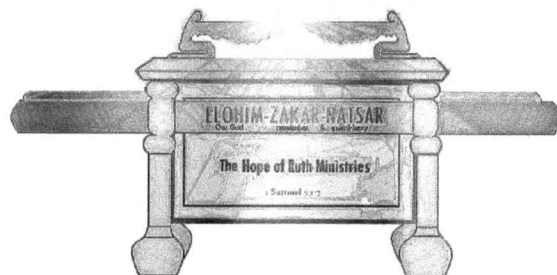

<u>Rebuilt Recovery Is a Ministry of The Hope of Ruth Ministries Church</u>

<u>Glorious Hope Publishing</u>

ISBN: 979-8-9852542-3-5 (Paperback)
Library of Congress Control Number: 2021922804

Glorious Hope Publishing
Hope of Ruth Ministries
307 Prentice Dr. New Carlisle, Ohio 45344
info@hopeofruthministries.com
www.hopeofruthministries.com

Thank you to the following people
who gave their ideas, hearts,
and lives into making this book possible.

Cindy Varghese

Summer Curtis

Alysha Allen

Justin Curtis

Annaka Schleinitz-Brooks

Jaycie Curtis

Camie Hawkins

Terri Allison

Contents

The Complete Rebuilt Series

Boxes and Symbols

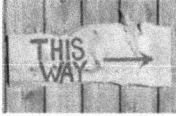

These boxes have thoughts or questions involving your coach.

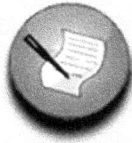

These boxes contain additional tasks for your journey.
Do not skip these tasks!

These boxes contain tips with additional information to help understand or implement the topic being discussed.

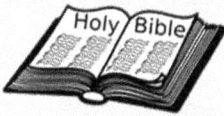

This icon indicates scripture important to understanding the current topic.

These boxes have important points for you to consider.

"These boxes contain interesting quotes"

Disclaimer

The information contained in the *Rebuilt for Life* (online course), *Rebuilt Recovery*, or *Rebuilt Website* is for general information purposes only. The content is not intended to be a substitute for professional advice, diagnosis, or treatment, rather it is intended as a supplement to it. Always seek the advice of your mental health professional or other qualified health provider with any questions you may have regarding your condition. It is your responsibility to inform your mental health professional that you are using a *Rebuilt* service to aid your recovery. Never disregard professional advice or delay in seeking it because of something you have read or heard in *Rebuilt* materials, website, or courses.

> If you are in crisis or have an emergency, call 911 immediately.
>
> **If you have suicidal thoughts, call the National Suicide Prevention Lifeline 1-800-273-TALK (8255) to talk with a skilled, trained counselor at a crisis center in your area.**
>
> **If you are located outside the United States, call your local emergency line immediately.**

Rebuilt coaches are not qualified counselors and do not take the place of certified professionals.

The information is provided by *The Hope of Ruth Ministries* and whilst we endeavor to keep the information up-to-date and correct, we make no representations or warranties of any kind, express or implied, about the completeness, accuracy, reliability, suitability, or availability with respect to the website, books, online course, the information, products, services, or related graphics contained on the internet or print materials for any purpose. Any reliance you place on such information is therefore strictly at your own risk.

In no event will we be liable for any loss or damage including without limitation, indirect or consequential injury, loss, or damage, or any injury, loss, or damage whatsoever arising from loss of life, relations, property, data, or profits arising out of, or in connection with, the use of the *Rebuilt* website, *Rebuilt for Life*, *Rebuilt Recovery*, or *Rebuilt Coaches*.

Every effort is made to keep the websites up and running smoothly. However, *The Hope of Ruth Ministries* nor *Rebuilt Recovery* takes no responsibility for, and will not be liable for, the coaches, website, software, or course being temporarily unavailable due to technical issues beyond our control.

COPYRIGHT NOTICE FOR SUPPLEMENTAL MATERIAL

All content on the website, *Rebuilt Recovery* books, and R*ebuilt For Life* online course is copyright protected. ©2020, 2021 Heather Phipps. All rights reserved. Limited rights are extended to *The Hope of Ruth Ministries*

Any redistribution or reproduction in part or totality of the contents in any form is prohibited, excluding Rebuilt worksheets available for download and extracts for your personal and non-commercial use only.

You may not, except with the express written permission of *The Hope of Ruth Ministries*, distribute, or commercially exploit the content. Nor may you transmit it or store it in any website or other form of electronic retrieval system.

EXTERNAL LINKS

Through the *Rebuilt* websites and courses, you may link to other websites, which are not under the control of *Rebuilt* or *The Hope of Ruth Ministries*. We have no control over the nature, content, and availability of such sites. The inclusion of any links does not necessarily imply a recommendation or endorse the views expressed within them.

Serenity Prayer

God, grant me the serenity
to accept the things I cannot change,
the courage to change the things I can,
and the wisdom to know the difference.

Living one day at a time,
enjoying one moment at a time;
accepting hardship as a pathway
to peace;

taking, as Jesus did,
this sinful world as it is,
not as I would have it;
trusting that You will make
all things right
if I surrender to Your will;

so that I may be reasonably happy
in this life
and supremely happy with You
forever in the next.

Amen.

Reinhold Niebuhr

Introduction to Book Three

Relationship with God

Having a relationship with God is vital to our faith. It is through relationship that we learn to understand the God we follow and know ourselves as individuals created in His image. It is only through our relationship with God that we can grasp who we are, identify lies about ourselves, and understand our purpose. Having a right relationship with God allows us to have healthy relationships with people and brings us to a place of biblical love for self. Confidence in God can give us confidence in ourselves—something we often lack.

To have confidence in yourself, you need to know the true source of your worth and value. In the last book, you took a step toward knowing yourself by examining what is in your heart. But to truly grasp your identity, you must know God. That will be the focus of this book.

In This Book

Blessings & Gratitude
In this chapter, you will learn how to change your focus from negative things in your life and discover how the Lord uses them for good, and you will learn to recognize hidden blessings.

Restoration
This chapter will focus on making amends and forgiving others. This helps put us in a right relationship with the Lord, releasing us from the burden of guilt and need for retribution, and relieving the pain in our heart for good.

Purpose
Your appreciation for life changes as you discover purpose and value through our God. This allows your confidence for your future to grow. You should not ask whether you are able. The real question is, do you believe God can make you able?

Loving Who You Are in Christ
You are worth everything God has for you because He has made you worthy. In this chapter, you will learn how you cannot love God or others without loving yourself. You will learn the difference between humility and living in humiliation. You will love the person God created you to be!

Identifying & Removing Lies
Who does God say you are? What is the truth you should hold, in contrast to the lies and labels you have been carrying through life? You are not what you do. You are not your past, your failures, or your mistakes. You are not the labels others have placed on you or the labels you place on yourself. So who are you? Do you trust the report of the Lord, which is truth and leads to life, or are you deceived by the report of the enemy, a lie that leads to death? Whose report will you believe?

Chapter Eleven

Blessings & Gratitude

Lesson 32 — Blessings

Serve the LORD with gladness! Come into his presence with singing! Know that the LORD, he is God! It is he who made us, and we are his; we are his people, and the sheep of his pasture. Enter his gates with thanksgiving, and his courts with praise! Give thanks to him; bless his name! For the LORD is good; his steadfast love endures forever, and his faithfulness to all generations. (Psalm 100: 2 – 5)

The Lord Makes Your Life a Blessing!

For I consider that the sufferings of this present time are not worth comparing with the glory that is to be revealed to us. (Romans 8:18)

In our inventory, we give a lot of attention to the negative things that happened in our lives. Here we look at how the Lord has used these situations to our good, and we recognize hidden blessings.

Rejoice always, pray without ceasing, give thanks in <u>all circumstances;</u> for this is the will of God in Christ Jesus for you. (1 Thessalonians 5:16 – 18)

It is easy to praise God when things are going well, but it is more difficult to praise Him in trials, pain, loss, and suffering. How do you react to life's difficulties? How do you respond to people failing you? Are you grateful through painful circumstances or when suffering loss?

Through him then let us continually offer up a <u>sacrifice of praise</u> to God, that is, the fruit of lips that acknowledge his name. (Hebrews 13:15)

I will offer to you the <u>sacrifice of thanksgiving</u> and call on the name of the LORD. (Psalm 116:17)

Scripture calls our praise a sacrifice. What makes gratitude and thanksgiving a sacrifice? The Hebrew word used for sacrifice is *zabach*, which means to slaughter. This raises the question: What does gratitude slaughter?

Praising the Lord slaughters self and destroys pride. When you give our gratitude to the Lord, you are sacrificing boasting in yourself to boast in Him. Gratitude sacrifices your right to self-pity. You must give up your attitude of grumbling and complaining, taking your attention off self, circumstance, and your right to "vent." Giving thanks slaughters our flesh to set our hearts on the goodness of the Lord. It is not possible to wallow in misery when you are praising the Lord.

Enter his gates with thanksgiving, and his courts with praise! Give thanks to him; bless his name! (Psalm 100:4)

Do not be anxious about anything, but in everything by prayer and supplication <u>with thanksgiving</u> let your requests be made known to God. (Philippians 4:6 – 7)

Do all things without grumbling or disputing. (Philippians 2:14)

Try this brief experiment
In your mind, say the alphabet and count to twenty simultaneously. It cannot be done. You may go back and forth between numbers and letters with super speed, but your **conscious mind** cannot think of both at the exact same moment. It is not possible to consider two thoughts at once, proving that while you are reflecting on praiseworthy things, negativity cannot inhabit your conscious thoughts.

The Mind of Christ

For who has understood the mind of the Lord so as to instruct him?
But we have the mind of Christ. (1 Corinthians 2:16)

Fill your mind with God's word. Fix your eyes on Him, and even in the most trying situations, you will see hope, truth, and a future of promise. **Negativity, fear, and worry are the fruit of a world deprived of God.**

God is good; He wills only good, and He works all things together for the good of those who love Him. He never has a gloomy outlook. **Therefore, a gloomy outlook does not unify us with God's mind and will.** God working all things for good means everything, even bad things, are beneficial for the believer. If you receive a situation as negative, you are not seeing it the way the Lord does. You have a corrupted perspective.

Negative thoughts are void of God's Word. The solution is more than attempting to speak God's Word into a circumstance to alter its outcome. It is knowing **God's mind** regarding your situations. It is **believing that truth and His purposes prevail** through every inconvenience and trial and in our lives. This is what it means to "fight the good fight of faith."

A Christian's confidence is knowing that God moves in everything.
A life surrendered, walking with God, cannot fail.

Identify Negativity

When you react to situations with worry, or have concern about the opinions or responses of others, are you trusting the Lord? Reactions that are fearful or riddled with anger and negativity show a place in your life where the truth of God's Word has not yet penetrated. **Use your negative thoughts and doubt** to discover areas devoid of His Word, to motivate your prayers, and to guide you into a deeper relationship with and greater trust of Him.

> ### Questions to Ponder
> 32.1) In what situations or areas of your life do you have a poor response? Where is there negativity in your thoughts?
>
> 32.2) How can you apply God's Word to the situations you identified?
>
> 32.3) Consider your negative situations, outlooks, and thoughts. In which areas do you recognize a need to grow in trust of the Lord?
>
> 32.4) How can you give praise to God in these situations?
>
> 32.5) In what areas are you still resentful of God? Where do you find it impossible to recognize anything good?

Lesson 33 — Seeing Life through New Eyes

At times, it is difficult to find God in life's trials. Have you ever wondered, "Where was God when I needed Him?" Scripture claims He **is** there, helping us overcome. The Lord does not hurt us, but sometimes His healing feels painful. Think of it as if you were going to the doctor with a broken bone. The doctor did not cause the injury, but for proper healing, he must rebreak and reset the bone. Likewise, the Lord does not cause our suffering, but the rebreaking required for healing can be painful.

He heals the brokenhearted and binds up their wounds. (Psalm 147:3)

For he wounds, but he binds up; he shatters, but his hands heal. (Job 5:18)

Why Do We Have Troubles?

Do you sometimes find it hard to understand why there is so much suffering in the world? Nowhere does Scripture say we will have an easy life. In fact, the Word tells us we enter God's Kingdom through trial and tribulation; but it also says the Lord will be with us in it.

Strengthening the souls of the disciples, encouraging them to continue in the faith, and saying that through many tribulations we must enter the kingdom of God.
(Acts 14:22)

Tests of faith strengthen us and increase our ability to persevere. Our weakness is the best display of God's power. Seeing the Lord work through difficulty teaches us to trust Him more.

Beloved, do not be surprised at the fiery trial when it comes upon you to test you, as though something strange were happening to you. (1 Peter 4:12)

So that the tested genuineness of your faith—more precious than gold that perishes though it is tested by fire—may be found to result in praise and glory and honor at the revelation of Jesus Christ. (1 Peter 1:7)

The enemy is not the only cause of our trials. Sometimes our flesh or other people's bad choices are the cause, and sometimes the Lord tests us. Whatever the cause, **God never wastes a situation or trial.** He uses it all to **keep us humble and transform our character.** The difficult things in life help us to grow. A test may come a short time after a victory, to strengthen an area we have overcome. The purpose is to go deeper into victory until we receive wholeness and perfection, standing firm in the Lord.

So to keep me from becoming conceited because of the surpassing greatness of the revelations, a thorn was given me in the flesh, a messenger of Satan to harass me, to keep me from becoming conceited. (2 Corinthians 12:7)

Count it all joy, my brothers, when you meet trials of various kinds, for you know that the testing of your faith produces steadfastness. And let steadfastness have its full effect, that you may be perfect and complete, lacking in nothing. (James 1:2 – 4)

The Lord uses hard situations to teach us about Him and His ways. He uses trials to show us truth, teach, and guide us, but He is gentle and disciplines us in love.

It is good for me that I was afflicted, that I might learn your statutes. (Psalm 119:71)

For the Lord disciplines the one he loves and chastises every son whom he receives.
(Hebrews 12:6)

How we handle trials may be an opportunity to make God known to the lost. When hardship weakens us, God's power is demonstrated in our lives.

I want you to know, brothers, that what has happened to me has really served to advance the gospel, so that it has become known throughout the whole imperial guard and to all the rest that my imprisonment is for Christ. And most of the brothers, having become confident in the Lord by my imprisonment, are much more bold to speak the word without fear.
(Philippians 1:12 – 14)

For the sake of Christ, then, I am content with weaknesses, insults, hardships, persecutions, and calamities. For when I am weak, then I am strong.
(2 Corinthians 12:9 – 10)

Trials may come simply because we follow Christ. Scripture says that a believer will share in the sufferings of Christ. The world will hate us for His name's sake, and we will suffer persecution, revilement, and false accusations. But Scripture also says that we have a glorious reward for our suffering.

Blessed are those who are persecuted for righteousness' sake, for theirs is the kingdom of heaven. Blessed are you when others revile you and persecute you and utter all kinds of evil against you falsely on my account. Rejoice and be glad, for your reward is great in heaven, for so they persecuted the prophets who were before you.
(Matthew 5:10 – 12)

God rewards us as we persevere and helps us overcome our suffering. **When God enters our mess**, He brings us through, and healing happens!

Many are the afflictions of the righteous, but the LORD <u>delivers him out of them all</u>.
(Psalm 34:19)

And after you have suffered a little while, the God of all grace, who has called you to his eternal glory in Christ, <u>will himself restore, confirm, strengthen, and establish you</u>.
(1 Peter 5:10)

The one who conquers and who keeps my works until the end, to him I will give authority over the nations.
(Revelation 2:26)

A God's Eye View of Your Life

When you look past your pain and discover the truth of Scripture in your trials, you will recognize the magnificence of the Lord. Only the Lord can show you His perspective on the events in your life. **The following tips and questions may aid your search for God's truth.**

- First, always test your beliefs against Scripture. If your thoughts do not line up with the **whole of Scripture**, they are not correct.

- Seek the Lord for His wisdom. Be open to hearing truth; the Lord will give understanding.

- Find the benefit resulting from the circumstance. What is the report of the Lord?

Questions to Ponder

33.1) Reexamine your heart check and inventory lists from God's perspective. Answer all six questions for each item mentioned in your inventory lists.

   1. What did you learn? What did the trial expose about your character?
   2. How was your faith tested?
   3. How did your character grow from the experience, or how could it have grown?
   4. How has the situation brought you to rely on God or increase your faith?
   5. How has God kept you from a greater harm in the situation?
   6. How has God improved your life or character (or the life or character of another) by allowing this to happen?

33.2) What good do you see from your trials? How can you give praise to God for the trials you have experienced in your life?

33.3) Write all the good and praises from the above answers in your Blessings Journal. *(Reference the homework below.)*

> ➤ **Begin a new "Blessings Journal" to keep a record of what the Lord has done in your journey and for your life.**
> ➤ **When you feel negative and discouraged, this journal will remind you of God's truth and provision.**
> ➤ **Pray your praises to the Lord!**

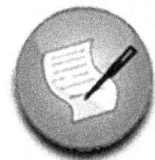

Chapter Twelve

Restoration

Lesson 34 — Forgiveness

During your inventory in Book Two, you found times that you hurt people, and times people hurt you. Although you gave your past pain to the Lord, **complete freedom** from anger, guilt, and fear requires that you release unforgiveness in your heart and make amends for your wrongs.

We will begin with forgiveness. Why start there? Sometimes, looking at your resentments toward others allows you to recognize your own wrongs. These situations may help you discover amends you need to make (though this is not always the case).

> ### Questions to Ponder
> 34.1) Define forgiveness. In your understanding, what does it mean to forgive someone?

Forgiveness Is Not …

Do you struggle to understand forgiveness? Society distorts the meaning, making true, biblical forgiveness a hard concept to grasp.

Do you find yourself replaying certain situations over and over in your mind, or do you feel like you must forgive someone repeatedly **for the same transgression**? If so, you may misunderstand forgiveness. Scripture commands believers to forgive, but many have no clue what that means. People often believe forgiveness means accepting someone's apology and not bringing the matter back up. This is not the definition of forgiveness. This cannot eliminate your pain; instead, it masks it. You need not forgive the **same event** multiple times. True forgiveness happens once per offense.

One common definition of forgiveness is a **decision to release resentful feelings** toward another who has harmed you, without condoning, excusing, or forgetting their wrong. Yet this definition is lacking. **How do you release resentful feelings without getting justice?** This definition bases forgiveness on **feelings**. With this notion of forgiveness, you create an **obligation** in your mind to no longer experience anger, even if it is entirely reasonable to have anger about a situation. **In reality, you are not forgetting the offense; you are attempting to forget what you** *feel* **about the offense.**

If your attempts at forgiving are ending resentment, you are probably understanding forgiveness in this way. Any trigger that reminds you of the wrong done to you brings back pain, and then you need to forgive again. It may take years for the resentment in your heart to dissipate, and this can cause a deeper, **repressed** resentment because you are pushing pain aside instead of addressing it.

Forgiveness Is …

Let us look at what is true in the false ideas of forgiveness discussed above. **Forgiveness is a choice** you make, but true forgiveness releases pain and resentment. You do not forget the offense, nor condone the wrong behavior. **Real forgiveness is a decision, not to release resentment, but to offer forgiveness**. People misunderstand forgiveness **because they do not understand the choice** they are making.

Releasing resentment is not forgiveness, rather is the result of forgiving.

11

The Greek biblical word for forgiveness is *aphesis,* which means dismissal, release, or pardon. We know a person should "pay" for harm they cause, and we have a right to justice. The demand in our heart for justice creates a burden of resentment and anger until restitution is made. **But it is also our God-given right to remedy the debt owed for harm another caused. Forgiveness is the remedy that cancels the debt.**

Consider a loan forgiveness program. The program "forgives" the owed debt and thereby cancels the debt. The lender can no longer ask you for the money because **the debt no longer exists.** It cleared as if paid in full, and the lender will never bring it back up again. The lender does not carry around a burden, waiting for the day you pay your debt.

In a similar way, actual forgiveness releases our right to retribution by giving the Lord our right to remedy the debt owed to us. This takes away our resentment as well. The Lord carries the burden of our retribution. **Collecting on the debt becomes His responsibility, and it is over for us.**

God wants this responsibility. Our sense of justice is corrupted by our emotions and sin nature. When we are harmed, we sometimes feel the consequence pales in comparison to the pain a person caused, wanting them to suffer more for their offense. When we are the offender, our efforts to resolve issues are sometimes lacking and disingenuous.

Because God is just, His forgiveness is based on the actions of the one needing forgiveness, but **our forgiveness cannot depend upon the actions of the one who hurt us.** Only God can remove a person's sin, and only His retribution is just. If the offender repents and comes to the Lord, He is right to forgive the offense. We can trust the Lord will work to bring the offender to repentance, and if they refuse, we can trust the Lord to handle it. **Either way, our forgiveness guarantees justice.**

The Rock, his work is perfect, for all his ways are justice. A God of faithfulness and without iniquity, just and upright is he. (Deuteronomy 32:4)

Forgiveness

God Himself models forgiveness for us. When we repent or turn away from our sin, He is faithful to forgive. Sin requires a penalty, and Jesus paid that debt. The wage of sin is death. **Jesus is like the loan forgiveness program that cancels our sin debt.** Our lives are the price we owe for our sins. **We pay the debt, one way or another.** If we decide to continue in sin, we pay the debt eternally. If we give our lives to the Lord, Jesus pays the price for us.

For the wages of sin is death, but the free gift of God is eternal life in Christ Jesus our Lord. (Romans 6:23)

The sting of death is sin, and the power of sin is the law. (1 Corinthians 15:56)

When we repent, the Lord separates us from our sin as far as the east is from the west, and He remembers it no more. Our debt collector no longer has the right to harass us, and sin loses its condemning power. When God forgives, He does not "forget" our sin; **He no longer remembers it.** What is the difference? God knows we committed the sin, but when he forgives, He no longer brings it to His memory to rehash or act on it. **God does not dwell on our past mistakes, and neither should we.** He helps us correct our mistakes and move forward. A sin forgiven is over. We need not continue to ask God's forgiveness for past wrongs.

Likewise, when we forgive someone for their wrongs to us, we do not need to remember or dwell on their sin. Yes, we know what happened, but we trust the Lord to make it right, and it opens the door to **restoration** of the relationship, *if the person is repentant* for their wrongs.

> *For I will be merciful toward their iniquities, and I will remember their sins no more.*
> *(Hebrews 8:12)*

> *As far as the east is from the west, so far does he remove our transgressions from us.*
> *(Psalm 103:12)*

Why Forgive?

➢ We forgive because we are forgiven.

> *Put on then, as God's chosen ones, holy and beloved, compassionate hearts, kindness, humility, meekness, and patience, bearing with one another and, if one has a complaint against another, forgiving each other; <u>as the Lord has forgiven you, so you also must forgive</u>.*
> *(Colossians 3:12 – 13)*

➢ As we forgive others is how we are forgiven.

> *For if you forgive others their trespasses, your heavenly Father will also forgive you, but if you do not forgive others their trespasses, neither will your Father forgive your trespasses.*
> *(Matthew 6:14 – 15)*

> *And whenever you stand praying, forgive, if you have anything against anyone, so that your Father also who is in heaven may forgive you your trespasses. (Mark 11:25)*

> *Judge not, and you will not be judged; condemn not, and you will not be condemned; forgive, and you will be forgiven. (Luke 6:37)*

> *Then his master summoned him and said to him, "You wicked servant! I forgave you all that debt because you pleaded with me. And should not you have had mercy on your fellow servant, as I had mercy on you?" And in anger his master delivered him to the jailers, until he should pay all his debt. So also my heavenly Father will do to every one of you, if you do not forgive your brother from your heart. (Matthew 18:32 – 35)*

➢ We are all sinners needing forgiveness.

> *If we say we have no sin, we deceive ourselves, and the truth is not in us. (1 John 1:8)*

➢ We forgive repeat offenses.

> *Then Peter came up and said to him, "Lord, how often will my brother sin against me, and I forgive him? As many as seven times?" Jesus said to him, "I do not say to you seven times, but seventy times seven." (Matthew 18:21 – 22)*

The Heart of Forgiveness

Scripture tells us that forgiveness is a genuine act of love. We are to love our enemies. Forgiveness begins with **pity**. What is the other person's situation? Pity for another does not excuse their actions; it is empathy for the pain in their hearts, which led them to hurt us. If we can understand the pain another has gone through, it is a step toward forgiving them.

Having a heart of **gratitude** makes it possible to forgive even devastating harm. If you are grateful for good resulting from a situation, forgiveness comes more easily. If you are grateful for the forgiveness you have received, it is easier to forgive another.

How Do I Forgive?

First, look at the harm and understand the situation. This does not justify another's actions, but it removes some of the emotional sting, allowing you to consider the whole picture.

- ➢ Start by asking yourself these questions:
    - ➢ What was the actual harm done?
    - ➢ Was the wrong intentional? What happened to cause the person to act that way? Is there room for pity?
    - ➢ Were their hurtful words or actions a response to something I did or said?
    - ➢ Was I correct in my handling of the situation? Were there wrongs on both sides?

- ➢ Next, release the offender from their debt of retribution.
    - ➢ Give it to the Lord and ask Him to take your pain and resentment. Allow the burden of justice to fall on His shoulders and not yours.

- ➢ Finally, expect God to be faithful and just, knowing that justice happens in His timing and may not be instantaneous.

Remember, **God is as patient with others as He is with you**. Have confidence that justice will come. If the offender repents and changes his way, then justice has come. If he does not repent, the Lord administers His justice. Either way, your pain is vindicated.

When Do I Forgive?

You should forgive as soon as possible. Otherwise, hurt festers inside and builds resentment in your heart. Forgiveness is for your freedom as much as, or more, than it is for the person you forgive.

Restoration

Forgiveness is not restoration. These are two separate things. To restore a relationship with someone requires that both parties understand the problem and walk in agreement. This is especially true when the person **continues to cause you the same harm**.

Reconciliation comes after a person shows repentance. Remember, repentance means the person changes how they treat you. **You can** forgive someone who is **not** repentant. However, you should **not restore a damaging relationship** that continues to hurt you. Restoration should happen only after the person repents. Reconciliation often requires rebuilding a relationship from a healthy starting point, or else the same harmful situations could repeat.

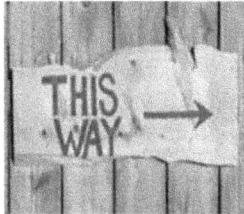

Make no effort at contact if harm could come to you or another person. It is not always necessary to tell someone you forgave them.

Ask your coach if you are unsure whether you should contact an offender or restore a relationship with someone.

Your coach is **not** permitted to tell you what to do in any given situation, but he or she may have additional insight that can help you make a wise decision.

Questions to Ponder

34.2) Do you understand forgiveness better since reading this lesson? Explain, in your own words, what forgiveness means, and how to forgive another.

34.3) Do you still hold resentment and unforgiveness toward anyone?

34.4) Write a letter to each person you need to forgive. Explain their actions and how you want to release them. *Do not give them the letters.* They are only meant to be a step to help you process your feelings.

34.5) Forgive any offenders and pray, giving the situation to the Lord. Give Him your burden, pain, and resentment. Relinquish your right to retribution to His perfect judgment and put your justice in His hands.

The next book goes into more detail about
restoring relationships and dealing with conflict.

Lesson 35 — Making Amends for Wrongs

In this lesson, you will examine and make amends for the wrongs you have done to others. Before you can confess your wrongs to another or to God, **you must admit them to yourself.**

> ### Questions to Ponder
>
> During your inventory, you made a list of people you have harmed by your words or actions. Has this list grown? Is there guilt in your heart not addressed in your list?
>
> **35.1) Add to your list any additional harms or recent harms you may have caused.**

Confess to Another and God

After identifying your wrongs, confess them. If you have not already done so, take the harms you caused others to your coach and pray for the Lord's forgiveness. Then your heart will be ready to make a genuine amends to the person whom you hurt if this is possible.

Why Should I Admit My Mistakes?

You may think because you did wrong years ago, there is no longer a reason to admit the mistake. Perhaps your actions cause you shame. No one wants to have to say, "I was wrong." For some people, admitting fault is terribly difficult. Yet making amends for your past wrongs is one of the most healing steps of your journey, not only for you, but also for the one to whom you apologize. We can never realize the full impact of our words and actions. Your apology may heal deep pain in a person's heart.

Admitting mistakes releases a burden from your shoulders that you may not even know you carry. It is a humbling experience, freeing you from the weight of guilt and regret. The heaviness of your secret sins lifts as you expose your wrongs to the light.

> *For when I kept silent, my bones wasted away through my groaning all day long. For day and night your hand was heavy upon me; my strength was dried up as by the heat of summer.*
> *(Psalm 32:3 – 4)*

> *Therefore, confess your sins to one another and pray for one another, that you may be healed. The prayer of a righteous person has great power as it is working.*
> *(James 5:16)*

What Does It Mean to Make Amends?

Making amends means taking responsibility for your wrong and attempting to make it right. Most often this is done with a letter or email containing a sincere, written apology and an admission of wrongs. In certain situations, this can also be a phone call or face-to-face visit.

Amends **may involve more than an apology**, such as restoring, repairing, or replacing an item you stole or damaged. Righting your wrongs is a biblical concept. The Lord can forgive you, but He still wants you to make it right and reconcile, with the one you harmed, if possible.

So if you are offering your gift at the altar and there remember that your brother has something against you, leave your gift there before the altar and go. First be reconciled to your brother, and then come and offer your gift.
(Matthew 5:23 – 24)

If a man steals an ox or a sheep, and kills it or sells it, he shall repay five oxen for an ox, and four sheep for a sheep. (Exodus 22:1)

Whoever conceals his transgressions will not prosper, but he who confesses and forsakes them will obtain mercy. (Proverbs 28:13)

What If I Am Uncertain about My Wrongs?

You may encounter times when people accuse you of wrongdoing, **but you were not in the wrong**. People sometimes make assumptions about your intentions from your past mistakes or their own past hurts. They may feel wronged if they dislike your actions or choices, or if your behavior calls out their own issues and wounds. **You cannot change how people feel about you or your actions.**

Examine a circumstance where you disagree with a person's determination of your guilt to confirm if there was an actual wrong, or if it was the other person's issue. Before making amends, ask yourself, "Was I wrong for this action? Could different actions or words have caused less harm?" **You should make amends if you caused genuine harm to another, but do not accept blame that does not belong to you.** If you are not wrong, maintain your innocence.

People may be oversensitive to what you say or do because of their own insecurity, fears, or hurts. You **can and should** consider their feelings. While it is not okay to accept blame for their misunderstandings, you may ease their concerns if you **clarify your intent or feelings**.

Sometimes we are oblivious to the fact that our words or actions harmed a person. You cannot change what you do not know. It is not beneficial to worry about wrongs you are not sure you committed. Scripture is clear: **We are to make amends when we become aware of the sin or harm we caused.** Ask the Lord to show you any wrongs you have done, then repent, forgive, and make amends.

If anyone sins, doing any of the things that by the Lord's commandments ought not to be done, though he did not know it, <u>then realizes his guilt</u>, he shall bear his iniquity. He shall bring to the priest a ram without blemish out of the flock, or its equivalent, for a guilt offering, and the priest shall make atonement for him for the mistake that he made unintentionally, and he shall be forgiven. It is a guilt offering; he has indeed incurred guilt before the Lord.
(Leviticus 5:17 – 19)

Risks and Responsibilities

A good amends speaks about growth, how you came to understand your wrong, the reason for your regret, and what you did or will do to correct it. **A genuine amends never includes a "but."** "I am sorry for this, but you made me so angry." Apologies that dig at the one to whom you are apologizing, or that attempt to shift the blame, are not genuine.

There is a risk when you admit your faults to someone you harmed. Not everyone will accept your apology or offer you forgiveness. This is okay. **You are correcting a wrong, not soliciting a response.** Your amends should be unconditional. Never base an apology on a person's acceptance of it. Clarify that your amends have **no expectations** attached.

People may have expectations after you make amends. They may wish to remain distant when you desire restoration, or they may want to restore the relationship when you believe it is unhealthy. Amends **may** open a door to reconciliation, yet sometimes it is not in your best interest, or theirs, to restore the relationship. **An apology does not obligate you to commit yourself to a toxic relationship.**

There is always the risk that a recipient of your amends may reject you and your apology. People sometimes cannot get past their own hurt. They may believe you are toxic to them and choose separation. There are many reasons a person is unable to hear your apology with the loving intent in which you wrote it. Do everything in your power to be at peace, but prepare for rejection.

If possible, so far as it depends on you, live peaceably with all. (Romans 12:18)

It is important to consider the possibility of harm from contacting a person. If it is possible that your amends will cause harm to you or others, **do not** approach the person. For example, a person may be unaware of the harm you caused, such as if you had judgmental or wrong thoughts about them. In this or any situation in which you cannot give an amends letter to the person you have wronged; you should still write the letter. Repent of your wrong thoughts or actions but share the amends letter only with God and your coach. Ask God's forgiveness and seek His wisdom about sharing the amends with the one harmed. Consult with your coach if you are unsure.

Questions to Ponder

35.2) Have you asked the Lord for forgiveness for all your wrongs? If not, do so now.

35.3) Are you prepared to express your regret for the harm you have caused?

35.4) Who may be harmed by your amends? Think about relationships that your letter might affect—*yourself, the one you harmed,* a *spouse, child, etc.*

35.5) Are there ways besides an apology to rectify some of your wrongs, such as restoring
or replacing something you took or damaged? If yes, list them.

35.6) Write a letter to each person to whom you need to make amends. Explain what you did to them, how you realized your wrong, and why you want to make it right.

    1. Explain that you have no expectation of a response to the letter.
      It is a no-strings-attached apology.

    2. Do not shift the blame. You are making an apology for your wrongs, not addressing their wrongs. Your apology should include no "but" statements.

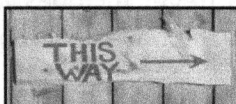

THIS WAY →   Do not approach someone, even by letter, if giving them an amends could cause you or another harm or put you in danger.

Chapter Thirteen

Purpose

Lesson 36 — Identity & Purpose

Have you ever wondered about your identity or purpose? Reading the Bible and calling on the Holy Spirit can help you discover your unique identity, purpose, and worth in Christ. The scriptures are more than generic statements for all followers; **they are specific to you**!

We have a future. We have an eternal purpose. We have hope. We have value.

Questions to Ponder

36.1) Do you struggle with knowing your identity in Christ? If yes, how?

36.2) Do you struggle to identify what makes you unique or special? Explain.

36.3) Do you struggle to know where you belong or to find a place to feel you "fit"?

36.4) What gives you value? Do you struggle to find your worth?

36.5) What do you believe is your purpose in life?

What Your Purpose Is NOT

Your purpose is not the "pursuit of happiness." **Happiness should not be a measure of success or value.** When you pursue the Lord's purpose for your life, **the result** includes happiness, but when your pursuit in life is merely to live happy, safe, and worry-free, you will find it to be a miserable existence. It is the trials in life—the sad moments and grief—which teach compassion, love, and strength of character, and which give our lives depth and meaning. No one likes hard times, but those living life to avoid difficulties can be destroyed when a crisis or trial causes their safe, happy, secure life to fail them.

> **"A life directed chiefly towards the fulfillment of personal desires will sooner or later always lead to bitter disappointment."**
>
> Albert Einstein in a Letter to T. Lee, January 16, 1954

When what you are living for fails you, where is your hope? You may become anxious or depressed and need to redefine what it is that makes life worth living. You need hope based in the Lord for a successful future. Knowing your true purpose never leaves you disappointed. God has unique plans for you, and His promises to give you both hope and a future will never fail.

For I know the plans I have for you, declares the Lord, plans for welfare and not for evil,
to give you a future and a hope. (Jeremiah 29:11)

Why Did God Create Us?

God was not lonely or vain when He created mankind, wanting someone to worship and adore Him. He did not desire servants or groundskeepers for the earth. God made the earth; He could care for it. God is not a control freak; He has every right to do as He wishes with His creation, **but He limited Himself** by giving us free will to make our own choices.

> *The God who made the world and everything in it, being Lord of heaven and earth, does not live in temples made by man, <u>nor is he served by human hands, as though he needed anything</u>, since he himself gives to all mankind life and breath and everything.*
> *(Acts 17:24 – 25)*

> So, why *would* He need us? The answer speaks volumes.
> God did *not* need us, He wanted us.

God created us to rule alongside Him. God's original intent for us is found in Genesis, when He created mankind **in His image and likeness** to fellowship and rule alongside Him.

> *Then God said, "Let us make man <u>in our image, after our likeness</u>. And let <u>them have dominion</u> over the fish … and over all the earth and over every creeping thing that creeps on the earth." (Genesis 1:26)*

> *Do you not know that <u>we are to judge angels</u>? How much more, then, matters pertaining to this life! (1 Corinthians 6:3)*

God created us to love us. "God is love" (1 John 4:8). Love, by definition, requires a recipient. God wants to overflow into us. God loved us even before we existed.

> *I have loved you with an everlasting love. (Jeremiah 31:3)*

God created us for relationship with Him. The depth and intimacy of the relationship God desires is apparent all throughout Scripture in the relationship language he uses: "father," "children," "husband," "bride," etc. God wants to share life with us.

> *<u>For your Maker is your husband</u>, the Lord of hosts is his name; and the Holy One of Israel is your Redeemer, the God of the whole earth he is called.*
> *(Isaiah 54:5)*

> *Let us rejoice and exult and give him the glory, <u>for the marriage of the Lamb</u> has come, and his <u>Bride</u> has made herself ready.*
> *(Revelation 19:7)*

> *And because you are sons, God has sent the Spirit of his Son into our hearts, crying, "<u>Abba! Father!</u>"*
> *(Galatians 4:6)*

He created us to share a divine nature with Him. God offers us everything we need to restore the divine nature lost in the garden, preparing us for eternal life with Him. Saved, we are **becoming a new creation**, able **to partake in his divine nature** and escaping the world's corruption (our sin nature).

His divine power has granted to us all things that pertain to life and godliness, through the knowledge of him who called us to his own glory and excellence, by which he has granted to us his precious and very great promises, <u>so that through them you may</u> <u>become</u> <u>partakers of the divine nature</u>, having escaped from the corruption that is in the world because of sinful desire.
(2 Peter 1:3 – 4)

What does it mean to "share a divine nature" with God? The answer takes us back to Genesis. In the beginning God created man in His image and likeness. Adam and his wife shared God's image and were like Him, **but that does not mean they were gods**.

Adam and his wife walked in the garden with God, in His image, clothed in His Spirit, His glory resting on them. God gave them authority over all the earth, allowing them to rule next to Him as perfect creations with a free will. **They shared God's divine nature, the character and virtue that He possesses**. It is a nature **built on sacrificial love**, a nature **void of sin**.

Adam and his wife **traded in this divine nature for a sin nature** when they chose to disobey God. There were two trees prominently displayed in the center of the garden: the Tree of Life, and the Tree of the Knowledge of Good and Evil, which led to "death." From the beginning mankind was offered the same choice we are offered today. We can choose life and live in God's ways, or we can choose to operate in our own knowledge of good and evil, a path that leads to death. What died the day they ate? It wasn't their bodies. Rather, the nature of who they were created to be died that day. **They transformed into sinners**.

Christ's sacrifice gave mankind the ability to make the same choice. Choose life by choosing God and **be transformed back into Christ's likeness**, restoring the divine nature that was lost, or choose death, eternal separation from God, by rejecting God's wisdom for our flesh.

God is our source of life. All things are of Him and exist through Him. The first couple's disobedience separated all people from the Lord. Like a plant cut away from its root that decays and dies, humans were separated from God, their source, by the power of sin. Sin corrupted the entire earth: people, plants, and animals. Because of sin we get sick, our bodies break down, and we die.

Adam and Eve lost the likeness of God when they sinned, trading in their divine nature for a sin nature. Every person's DNA was in the first couple. When they fell, all of humanity fell with them, the seed corrupted. Therefore, the power of sin is at work in each of us from conception.

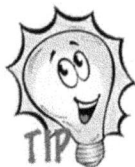

When we understand that we were created to be loved by God Himself, we can see that our **first purpose** is to have relationship with Christ. As that relationship grows, the Lord transforms our heart into His own likeness, restoring the likeness to the divine nature that was lost through sin. **This life is like boot camp training for our eternal purpose**, to rule and reign with Christ!

36.6) How does knowing why God created us help us to understand our purpose?

36.7) How would you define God's main purpose for mankind, and for you personally?

His Plan and Purpose

And we know that God causes all things to work together for good to those who love God, to those who are called according to His purpose. For those whom He foreknew, He also <u>predestined</u> to become conformed to the image of His Son, so that He would be the firstborn among many brethren; http://biblehub.com/romans/8-30.htm*and these whom He predestined, He also called; and these whom He called, He also justified; and these whom He justified, He also glorified. What then shall we say to these things? If God is for us, who is against us?*
(Romans 8:28 – 31)

God orchestrates all history for the benefit of those who are His. He knew our beginnings, our choices, and our ending before we ever were. Believers have a promise that He will redeem every moment of our life, forming it into good for us and others whom He has called.

➤ **Our purpose is to do His will.** You are predestined, meaning God planned you for this exact moment of time, so He could save all who would be saved. He plans to prosper each one of us, giving us a future and hope. The first and most important of those plans is to **draw us into proper relationship with Him** and transform us into His likeness.

➤ **Our purpose is love.** To be created in "God's likeness" means we shared God's attributes. It makes sense, then, that to restore our Christlikeness, we must be a people who love. Scripture states that we know followers of Jesus by their love for one another.

Your Life Has Purpose

God also has a specific plan and purpose for your life as an individual. Although God does require you to lay down your sin nature, he does not require you to give up who you are; **He made you unique to fulfill his purpose.** He equips each person with talents and gifts, whether we believe in Jesus or have any relationship at all with God.

We choose how we use our gifts. Those in the world who lack a relationship with Jesus often use their gifts and talents to prosper their own lives and fulfill the desires of their flesh. Those who live by the Spirit will take all that they are—their talents, gifts, and desires—and wrap them around the Lord to use for His glory and Kingdom purposes.

> (!) You may find that God's mission is not the same as what you envisioned for your life. **Be assured**, however, that **His mission for you will fill you with joy**. You will experience satisfaction and fulfillment when you walk in His ways!

Consider ranks in the Army: a private has the least authority, and a general has the most authority. No other rank answers to the private, except when the general gives the private a mission. The private then carries the same authority as the general regarding that mission. **All** other ranks submit to him. **God is your general.** Everything submits to His authority, and when you are fulfilling His mission, you operate with His authority.

When we allow God to move **through** our gifts and talents, **we succeed**. God gives us gifts to help us **achieve the calling and purpose He has** for us. When we use our God-given abilities to carry out **His** plans, we cannot fail, because we have the power and authority of the Almighty God behind us.

"If you live outside the will of God, if you act against it, then you will live and act with the authority of a private, which is to have no authority. But if you live inside the will of God, if you follow the directives of God, if you carry out His assignment, if you set your course on fulfilling His mission, then you will live in the authority of God. Then every rank in this universe must yield to your steps, every door must unlock, and every gate must open. So, make it your aim to live your life wholly in the will of God. Find your mission and fulfill it. … And you will walk in the power and authority of the Almighty."

Jonathan Cahn, *The Book of Mysteries* (2016), "The Private and the General", p.133

Questions to Ponder

36.8) What do you think success in God's Kingdom looks like?

36.9) How does this differ from what the world sees as success?

36.10) What are your plans, your goals, dreams, and desires for the future? Seek the Lord about your purpose.

36.11) Can you imagine God prospering you in these pursuits? How?

36.12) Proverbs 19:21 says, "Many are the plans in the mind of a man, but it is the purpose of the LORD that will stand." What does this passage mean to you? Explain.

36.13) Are you okay with God's plans for your life, even if they differ from what you think you want? How will following His plans affect you?

Chapter Fourteen

Loving Who You Are in Christ

Lesson 37 — Defining Love

How Important Is Love?

Love is everything. Without love we are nothing. We are able to love as a result of receiving God's love. We respond to His love and express our love for God by keeping His commandments. God's commandments are to love Him and to love others as ourselves. To overflow love into another, we must receive God's love. If our love for ourselves does not come from God, our attempts to love others will arise from a selfish need to fill an empty place in our heart. The more we love ourselves as God wants us to, the more we can love others as ourselves.

And if I have prophetic powers, and understand all mysteries and all knowledge, and if I have all faith, so as to remove mountains, <u>but have not love, I am nothing</u>. (1 Corinthians 13:2)

We love because he first loved us. (1 John 4:19)

➤ How do we love God? Jesus said the way we love Him is by keeping His commandments.

If you love me, <u>you will keep my commandments</u>. (John 14: 15)

Whoever has my commandments and keeps them, he it is who loves me. And he who loves me will be loved by my Father, and I will love him and manifest myself to him. (John 14:21)

➤ All God's commandments derive from these two: Love God and love others as yourself.

"Teacher, which is the great commandment in the Law?" And he said to him, "<u>You shall love the Lord your God</u> with all your heart and with all your soul and with all your mind. This is the great and first commandment. And a second is like it: <u>You shall love your neighbor as yourself</u>. On these two commandments depend all the Law and the Prophets. (Matthew 22:36 – 40)

➤ We are to love God, but to love God we must obey His commandment to love others.

Anyone who does not love does not know God, because God is love. (1 John 4:8)

If anyone says, "I love God," and hates his brother, he is a liar; for he who does not love his brother whom he has seen cannot love God whom he has not seen. (1 John 4:20)

Jesus commands us to love our neighbor (others) **as we love ourselves**. The more we love ourselves, the better we love others, and the more our love for God shows. The question then becomes, **"What does it mean to love yourself?"**

Loving Myself vs. Humility

You may wonder how you can have humility and love yourself. **Humility is not thinking less of yourself, it is thinking more of God.** It is building up another's qualities, not bragging about your own. It is esteeming others, giving them recognition before taking the glory for yourself. **Humility is not putting yourself down or treating yourself poorly.**

To gain more clarity about this, let us define what humility is and is not.

Humility is not:

- Thinking you are bad

- Seeing yourself as less valuable or worthy than another person

- Feeling or acting as if you do not matter

- Feeling or acting as if you are not good enough

The previous list describes, not humility, but humiliation. Humiliation actually masks pride. When we act in humiliation, we want others to feed our pride in order to combat our insecurity. People who live in humiliation often behave pridefully, as if they are secure and confident, but they do this to hide their insecurity.

Humility is:

- Seeing yourself honestly, **not as more or less** than you are

- Knowing that without God you can do nothing, but with God you can do all things

- Esteeming others over yourself **without** regarding them as having greater worth

- Feeling or acting as if you do not matter

- Feeling or acting as if you are not good enough

- Giving others respect, admiration, and honor **before** accepting it for yourself

- Knowing that you have value that comes, **not from yourself, but from God**

- Living a life led by the Lord and **dying to your own will**

Humility is the first step in loving yourself because humility is where God changes your heart. Here is a saying to remember when you are struggling in your relationship with God: **Pride prevents progress.** For God to change your life, you must have the attitude that He knows better than you.

Questions to Ponder

37.1) Do you act in humiliation or in humility?

37.2) How has your pride prevented God from making progress with you in your journey?

37.3) When looking at yourself, do you like or dislike what you see?

37.4) Can you say that you love yourself? Describe what you feel about yourself.

We tend to act from self-preservation when we believe we are undeserving of love, have a poor self-image, or carry deep shame. **This makes it impossible to show selfless love** to others. When strongholds like fear or anger dictate our thinking, they filter how we see others. **We often assume people think and act the same way we would in any given situation.** When we are stuck in shame and wrong thoughts about ourselves, we are more likely to misjudge others' motives as well. We struggle to love others properly because we "love" them **out of our own need** for love instead of a desire to give of ourselves to them.

Our ability to love our neighbor is dependent on how we value ourselves.
With a godly view of ourselves, we are able to give and receive God's kind of love!

Love Defined

People tend to abuse the word *love*. People can also abuse others in the name of love, or use "love" to manipulate others for their own selfish ends. When we have difficulty trusting in other people's love, we will struggle to trust God's love. We may see God as either a harsh judge or uninvolved. However, Scripture says God is **love**. If we cannot understand God's love, we will never have a correct perception of God.

Everybody agrees love is good, but we do not agree on what love is. **It is impossible to accept or display a love we do not understand.** Today, many people equate love with gushy emotions, selfish desires, or sexual intimacy. I love my friend. I love pizza. I love my first crush … and then next year, I love another. We have deeper forms of love also, such as the love for our children, spouse, parents, and God. These experiences are all different, yet we use the same word, love, to describe them all. Love has become very confusing.

The two Hebrew words used in the Bible to express love are *ahava* and *chesed*, and these words give a clearer understanding of God's love. ***Ahava* and *chesed* display attributes of God.** The writers of the New Testament Greek used the word ***agape*** to attempt to capture the meaning of these two Hebrew words.

CHESED: This word can express love from God to people, or between people.
- Translations describe *chesed* as **loving-kindness, mercy, steadfast love, compassion, loyalty, goodness, great kindness, favor, and loyalty.** It is an **unfailing, everlasting, steadfast, and loyal love**, an **eternal faithfulness** or **devotion**.

- *Chesed* is **unselfish love**, and it is proven in actions performed **with no thought of "what's in it for me?"** The expression of this kind of love is **not dependent on your mood or what you feel.**

- *Chesed* is **a love that surpasses your own hurts.** It overcomes the harm people do through their words, their sin, and their betrayal. *Chesed*'s **compassion motivates** us to extend grace, mercy, and forgiveness.

- *Chesed* is more than charity *(tzedakah)*. It is an **excess or overflowing** of kindness, going beyond what is required or expected. *Chesed* **produces** abundant, extravagant giving and acts of charity, mercy, and kindness toward someone in a greater measure than they **deserve.**

The Pharisees performed acts of charity *(tzedakah)*; Jesus expected love *(chesed)*.

AHAVA: This word represents our love toward God. It is selfless, not dependent upon what He does for us. We express this love through action, and therefore it is **a choice**.

- o *Ahava* is both a noun and a verb representing both the actions of love and the feeling of love. It represents a feeling **because** of an action, not an action as the **result** of a feeling.

- o The root word *ahav* means **to give**. Therefore, this love **is not something that happens to you**, but something that **comes from you**. Your act of giving generates *ahava*, regardless of whether the giving is of your affection, time, or resources.

- o *Avaha* should be **the intent** behind our thoughts, words, and actions, and our motivation for obedience in response to Jesus' command: "If you love Me, you will keep My commandments" (John 14:15).

AGAPE: This is the most used and important word for love found in the New Testament.

- o It is the closest word in the Greek to express the Hebrew concept of selfless love.

- o This love relates to what God prefers, to his ways, as "God is love" (1 Jn 4:8,16), and therefore it **relates to righteousness**. The greatest act of love was Jesus giving His life to cover the sins of mankind and make us righteous in His sight!

These words for love create a picture of the love Jesus calls us to have for God, our neighbors, and ourselves. **In none of these words do we find the connotation of a feeling creating love.** We can love others without feeling it. It is often after we exhibit love that we experience the resulting emotion. This is easier to understand when we think about loving other people or God, but **more difficult when we think about loving ourselves**.

> ⓘ **QUICK FACT**
>
> Many people are familiar with the Greek word *agape* used to describe love in the New Testament, but did you know there are two other Greek words occasionally used to express love?
>
> *Storge* describes love for family, and *phileo* describes the love you would have for a close friend. *Phileo* is affection based in feelings, or it can be a sentiment toward an object. *(I love pizza.)*
>
> **These words do not speak to a godly or sacrificial love.**

Questions to Ponder

37.5) What are the attributes of a biblical love?

37.6) How has your understanding of the nature and expression of love changed after reading this lesson?

37.7) What attributes of God can you identify as love?

37.8) What parts of Scripture do you find difficult to accept as God's love?

37.9) For each thing you mentioned in answering the previous question, describe how each could be an act or expression of God's love.

37.10) Describe how you can love yourself without "feeling it".

Why Righteousness?

Is it love to enable someone to continue in destructive sin? Of course not! **Love corrects and protects.** It is that very question that leads us to know that **every** attribute of God is love. His justice, authority (law), and judgment are love as much as his grace and mercy are love. It can be easier to accept God's discipline for someone who hurt you than to accept His discipline for yourself. The Lord compares his reproof to a father disciplining His son. While it is uncomfortable, He intends it to help us mature.

> *My son, do not despise the LORD's discipline or be weary of his reproof, for the LORD*
> *reproves him whom he loves, as a father the son in whom he delights.*
> *(Proverbs 3:11 – 12)*

> *Have you forgotten the exhortation that addresses you as sons? My son, do not regard*
> *lightly the discipline of the Lord nor be weary when reproved by him. For the Lord*
> *disciplines the one he loves and chastises every son whom he receives. It is for discipline*
> *that you have to endure. God is treating you as sons. For what son is there whom his*
> *father does not discipline? If you are left without discipline, in which all have*
> *participated, then you are illegitimate children and not sons.*
> *(Hebrews 12:5 – 7)*

A Heavenly Father's Love

God designed the family to teach us about Himself and about love. In a fallen world, however, our families are flawed, sometimes with significant dysfunction. Since no one has a perfect family, **we must not attribute their flaws and failures to God**. His Word can make up where families fall short. God is the perfect father, teaching and helping us to grow, but **He is not abusive or cruel**. He never leaves us to fight our battles alone, but stands by our side. His discipline is for our welfare and not to harm us. **He convicts us of our sin, like a good father** who instructs his son about right and wrong, **and He is our safety net**, so the consequences of our sins do not destroy us.

> *"Do not fear, O Jacob My servant," says the LORD, "For I am with you; For I will*
> *make a complete end of all the nations to which I have driven you, but I will not*
> *make a complete end of you. I will rightly correct you, for I will not leave you*
> *wholly unpunished." (Jeremiah 46:28)*

God's discipline is not punishment for the sake of punishment. Discipline may include a natural consequence, but it is designed to teach us and help us grow into wholeness and perfection, preparing us for eternity. God's discipline is always out of love and always for our benefit.

> *Count it all joy, my brothers, when you meet trials of various kinds, for you know that*
> *the testing of your faith produces steadfastness. And let steadfastness have its full*
> *effect, that you may be perfect and complete, lacking in nothing.*
> *(James 1:2 – 4)*

Questions to Ponder

37.11) Describe God as a father.

37.12) Describe the love you received from your parents as a child. How was their love a good representation of God's love?

37.13) In what ways was the parenting you received as a child a poor representation of God's love?

37.14) How is your love for your spouse teaching you about a loving relationship with Christ as His bride? *(If you are not married, how can you imagine love for a spouse teaching you about this relationship with Christ?)*

37.15) How can your marriage *(or future marriage)* be a bad example of relationship with Christ?

Lesson 38 — Addressing Shame

Questions to Ponder

38.1) Do you *feel* like you love yourself?

38.2) How do you treat yourself with love?

38.3) Think about the definitions of love in the previous lesson. Based on these definitions, how can you love yourself better?

Are You Bad?

Surely I was brought forth in iniquity; I was sinful when my mother conceived me. (Psalm 51:5)

Among whom we all once lived in the passions of our flesh, carrying out the desires of the body and the mind, <u>and were by nature children of wrath, like the rest of mankind.</u>
(Ephesians 2:3)

Do you ever feel confused when you try to think of yourself as righteous, justified, or a saint? Would you call yourself "good"? How do you reconcile the idea that you are righteous when you know your sinful thoughts and ways? If you are always confident in your righteousness, you are in the minority. Maybe you compare yourself to "better" Christians, wear a Christian mask, or fall short of your expectations. When you examine your heart and see the sin and wickedness within, it may be difficult to "feel" righteous, **yet Scripture says our faith is our righteousness and our justification is by the sacrifice of Jesus**.

Defining Good and Bad

God did not design good to exist apart from Him. He is good, and apart from Him nothing can be good. **Therefore, evil is what exists in the absence of God, and sin is the force which perpetuates evil.** The evil, hardship, and destructive force of decay and death were **not** God's design for this world. These things resulted from sin entering the world. The same pattern that ensnared Eve in the garden continues today, as shown in the book of James. No one is exempt from sin.

But each person is tempted when he is lured and enticed by his own desire. Then desire when it has conceived gives birth to sin, and sin when it is fully grown brings forth death.
(James 1:14 – 15)

Eve had distorted thoughts when the enemy **tempted her** to disobey God. Her **desire for wisdom enticed** her, and then the desire **gave birth to her plan of action**: eating the fruit. The sin committed **brought forth death**, or separation from God. Mankind lost their divine nature, exchanging it for an "evil nature"—our sin nature.

God knitted each of us together in the womb as a perfect creation, yet we are tainted at conception by sin's power. God did not create wicked people. He created people who became wicked because they have a corrupting sin nature. **Only God can change it.**

There is good news, though: **God knew this would happen and developed a backup plan,** even before laying the foundations of the earth. Jesus agreed to pay the penalty for our sin with His own blood, thus removing the separation of man from God, bringing life, and allowing us to regain fellowship with God. We become clean from our sin; our divine nature restored. As we head into our eternal existence, we will receive a new, incorruptible body, unaffected by the power of sin.

What does this mean to you? By accepting Christ as your Lord and Savior, you gave God permission to **change your nature.** In Christ, you must no longer carry the label of bad, the label of shame. You are a **redeemed saint** living in an evil world with a **nature prone to sin.** You will never be perfect while living on this earth, but your life in Christ will show fruit of **His likeness.** We have a promise that one day we will be perfect and complete, lacking in nothing, if we can persevere. **Becoming Christlike is a life-long process.**

> ### Questions to Ponder
> 38.4) In what areas of your life do you feel inadequate?
>
> 38.5) How do you handle your mistakes?
>
> 38.6) In what ways do you allow past failures and mistakes to define you?
>
> 38.7) How should your thoughts regarding your sin and shame change?

Labels

From our earliest moments we want to define things. Born with curiosity about our world and ourselves, we look to others to understand our place. We begin life mimicking behaviors and actions we see, attempting to discover our limits and our identity.

This process covers us with labels. As our vocabulary grows, the label game begins. Every experience, mistake, assumption, and influence adds a label. We strive to be special and unique, to excel, and to stand out because we want to define our labels. These labels become our identity.

Identity labels

We project the identity labels we want others to see in us—labels like powerful, secure, and creative. These **identity labels are our "walls."** We cover ourselves in these walls to give us a sense of self-worth and value. We seek people with similar walls to find belonging. Identity labels define how our mind perceives the person we **should be.**

As we go through life, **people attempt to modify our labels with their own.** (You are pretty, ugly, the love of my life, a brat ...) The negative labels people and our experiences place on us become shame in our hearts. Shame creates more shame as our own minds betray us, reinforcing this distorted picture of ourselves.

Shame Labels

The Insults and condemnation other people claim for us produce shame labels. These labels may also come from expectations others want us to meet, or from praise and flattery for an image we cannot maintain. Shame labels shape how our mind perceives the person **we are.** We bury shame labels deep beneath our walls (our identity labels) to keep them hidden.

The way others treat us and their words are a powerful influence guiding our perception of our worth. People's words and our circumstances continually reinforce this skewed perception. The enemy takes advantage, whispering lies that we are not enough: not good enough, not smart enough, not attractive enough, not successful enough. We then end up comparing ourselves to others or to some unachievable expectations we decide we must meet.

Our insecurities drive us to be better and better, but we always seem to fall short of our "enoughs." This reinforces the labels others have given us. We then make a choice to either accept those labels or combat them with our own. **Yet the truth is that none of these labels define us.** The only accurate labels are the ones given to us by the Lord, and therefore, believing the label lies of ourselves and others, leads to shame.

What is shame? We all make mistakes and have varying degrees of guilt. We do wrong, apologize, try to make it right, and then move on. However, sometimes our mistakes reinforce negative beliefs we have about ourselves. **We exchange the guilt of *doing* something bad for a deep-seated belief that we *are* something bad.** This is the shame that keeps us defeated.

Words influence how we understand our identity, but our labels do not define us. **They are just a sticker on the outside of the package with a misleading ingredients list**, giving us a false view of our worth. If we believe our labels, we will become either pumped up in pride, or waste away in shame and feelings of worthlessness.

Questions to Ponder

38.8) What words or actions of your parents or caregivers when you were a child influence your thoughts or reactions now?

38.9) What words or events from your early childhood sent you positive messages?

38.10) What words or events from your early childhood reinforced your shame?

38.11) Consider your teen and adult years. How have events and words affected your internal belief about your worth?

38.12) List the identity labels that define you.

38.13) List the shame labels that define you.

38.14) Reflect again about the labels that define you. Do you see anything new or recent?

38.15) What experience caused each shame or identity label you listed?

38.16) Looking back on the labels you have believed throughout your life, how have your shame and identity labels influenced your responses?

You are *not* what you do.
You are *not* your past, your failures, or your mistakes.
Only the Lord defines your identity.

Lesson 39 — Your Path Defines You

How Do You *Know* Who You Are Beneath Your Masks and Labels?

All people are:

Created for relationship with God

Created for love and to love

Created for righteousness

People have a choice:

Choose to accept and become the person they were created to become

Choose to pursue self and cling to their sin nature

The person we desire to become shows our heart, the genuine person existing deep in our soul. We may not like our actions, but **our actions do not define us; our path defines us.**

Our Path Defines Us

If we choose to **satisfy our sin nature**, rejecting God's ways, then we travel on **a path of destruction, and the enemy gets to define our identity**. If we choose **God's path** and pursue righteousness, then **He defines our identity**.

For example, a man whose deepest desire of his heart is to become rich or powerful might use any method to achieve that desire. He may steal, cheat, manipulate, or use people to reach his goals, feeling justified in doing so. **His desires and motives** are for self and reveal who he truly is and the path of life he has chosen.

Another man may desire wealth, but the deepest desire of his heart is to help people and invest into the lives of others. His desire for riches is for investment into his community. He strives for that success, but his heart's desire is to be someone who loves people. His desires and motives also show his true identity and a path after the heart of God.

Nearly everyone desires success, but not everyone defines success the same way. Success to some looks like the world: prosperity, notoriety, position, power. For others it looks like a happy family, raising successful kids, bringing people to know Jesus, or serving and investing in the lives of others. How you define success is another important key to defining who you are. **It is not the desire, but the motive in your heart fueling the desire which reveals your path.** When your motives line up with God's will, you can be assured you are on His path.

Questions to Ponder

39.1) **Imagine what the perfect person would be like? Describe details of his or her character, personality, and abilities.** (Your perfect person would be one you can admire, respect, and want to be like—someone you would become if it were possible. Note: this is hypothetical. No one is perfect.)

39.2) Is the person you described worthy of your love? Is it someone you want to become?

39.3) Do you think you can become like this person? Why or why not?

39.4) Define the deepest desires of your heart regarding the character and identity you desire for yourself. Be honest.

39.5) How do you define success for your life?

39.6) Narrow your definition of a successful life to one achievement that gives your life value and meaning.

39.7) Describe the path in life that you have chosen.

Good News

Your picture of a perfect person reflects the person you desire to become. **Your perfect person reflects the values of your heart!** This person is inside you, waiting to come out.

Sometimes our beliefs of what makes someone "good" are based on other people's perceptions of the right way to be in life. Parents, teachers, role models, and friends have instilled in us some of their beliefs.

If your perfect person does not line up with the deep desires of your heart, you may be listening to a voice that is not your own. For example, if your dad raised you to never show weakness, your perfect person may have characteristics of safety and strength, never showing emotion or pain. However, when you defined your deepest desires, you may have included empathy for others. You cannot have empathy for someone without emotions. The person in this example is double minded in this area. He would need to examine what he really feels and believes apart from what others have told him or modeled for him. Before you can determine who you really are as a person, or if your beliefs are right or wrong, you must sort through and discover **what you think for yourself.**

> The character and personality of your perfect person,
> how you define success, and the spiritual path you choose define you.
> *In Christ, this is the person God created you to be, and this is a person you can love. Strive with the Lord to become that person!*

39.8) If your perfect person does not match up to the deepest desires of your heart, how are they different?

39.9) Do you have some ways of thinking that are not your genuine beliefs, but the beliefs of another? What are they?

Questions to Ponder

39.10) Examine your answers to all the questions from this lesson. Use the characteristics of your perfect person, your definition of success, and the path you have chosen for life to write what life would look like as your perfect person.

39.11) Read your answer to the previous question. This description describes who your heart says you are. What does this say about your identity, potential, and purpose?

Find three people whose opinion matters most to you and have each one list everything they like about you, especially referring to your character. Each person should seal their lists in an envelope. Do not look at what they wrote ... yet.

Chapter Fifteen

Identifying & Removing Lies

Lesson 40 — Who You Are in Christ

In Christ, we have a new identity. As we discovered in the last lesson, we are transforming into a new creation. So, what is this new identity? Where does our worth come from? You have identified your walls (identity labels) and your shame (lies you believe about yourself); now it is **time to reveal your real label**.

The Lord gives you a seal, which is your genuine label. The Holy Spirit confirms your seal, bearing witness with your own spirit that you belong to Him. Then He begins transforming you into the righteous new creation promised by your faith in Christ.

And it is God who <u>establishes us</u> with you in Christ, and has <u>anointed us</u>, and who has also <u>put his seal on us</u> and given us <u>his Spirit</u> in our hearts <u>as a guarantee</u>. (2 Corinthians 1:21 – 22)

The following are just a few of the scriptures that describe our identity in Christ:

- *"Do you not know you are <u>God's temple</u> and that God's Spirit dwells in you?"* *(1 Corinthians 3:16)*

- *"No longer do I call you servants, for the servant does not know what his master is doing; but <u>I have called you friends</u>." (John 15:15)*

- *"But to all who did receive him … he gave the right to become <u>children of God</u>." (John 1:12)*

- *"But you are a <u>chosen race, a royal priesthood, a holy nation, a people for his own possession</u>, that you may proclaim the excellencies of him who called you out of darkness into his marvelous light." (1 Peter 2:9)*

- *"Therefore, if anyone is in Christ, he is <u>a new creation</u>." (2 Corinthians 5:17)*

In Christ we are secure, sealed, protected, and sustained
despite our circumstances or past sins.

How does God see you? Scripture tells us everyone has sinned and fallen short of the Glory of God. Why would God, the creator of heaven and earth, want to be your friend? How does that happen?

God hates sin because it separates us from Him. He is holy and righteous, and He cannot be with evil. How can God look at us, people who do evil, and claim we are righteous? In the Old Testament, He even called David, an adulterer and murderer, a man after His own heart. How can this be?

God sees our final product. He is the Alpha and Omega, the beginning and the end. He sees the past, future, and all points in between. We go through life as if traveling a straight line in front of us, only seeing one step ahead and everything behind us. God, however, sees life from a full perspective of history. He has a bird's-eye view of our lives. He knows the person He created us to be and the person we will become. **Therefore, we look at ourselves and see one thing, but God looks at us and sees something completely different!**

The Lord fixes His eyes on who we are becoming, not who we are now.

We see ourselves:	He sees us:
In turmoil	Peaceful
Broken	Healed
Rejected	Chosen
Without a voice	God's ambassador
Guilty and condemned	Righteous and justified
Fearful	Faithful
Trapped	Free
A mistake	Ordained with purpose
A failure/loser	Successful/victorious
Worthless	Valuable
Weak	Strong
No future	With a future and hope
Ugly/disabled/diseased	Fearfully and wonderfully made

We Are a Work in Progress

What does the process of creating a prized sculpture look like? The sculpture starts out as nothing more than a lump of clay. The sculptor begins shaping the clay. You can only catch a hint of what he is creating. As it nears completion the clay looks more like the finished product, but it is still flawed. You cannot see its flawless beauty until the sculptor completes his work. Likewise, we are incomplete, still in the molding process, with the potential to become glorious!

Imagine if the lump of clay spoke and had free will. What if it said, "No, I am ugly, I am only clay?" What if the clay became so set on its flawed appearance that it refused to allow the sculptor to work? It would never transform. It would forever remain an ugly lump of clay.

If you created a masterpiece, would you throw your work away? Would that masterpiece have value? You are God's masterpiece, a lump of clay in your maker's hands. With every work God does in your heart, you are becoming closer to the image of perfection that God promises for you, a beautiful sculpture in His hands, in the likeness of your creator. He gives another promise, too: He will complete the work He began in you! Focus on the person you are becoming and leave the shame of the past in the past.

And I am sure of this, that he who began a good work in you will bring
it to completion at the day of Jesus Christ. (Philippians 1:6)

Discerning Truth and Deception

This world disguises bad as good and good as bad. If Satan walked up to you looking evil, you would reject him. Instead, **he disguises his lies as truth**, feeding off your self-doubt and insecurity. His lies are reinforced by the harsh words and actions of others and validated as you make comparisons and try to measure up to false standards. You lie to your soul with each thought that screams you are not good enough. Who is good enough?

But when they measure themselves by one another and compare
themselves with one another, they are without understanding.
(2 Corinthians 10:12)

Sometimes the deception you believe **is not lies masked in a disguise of truth, but a truth hidden by a lie**. Like a forest in the winter, every tree appears dead. The teeming life of the forest is hidden away, waiting for the spring. Walking in the woods on a winter day, the appearance of death is stark. For a person unfamiliar with the seasons, it may seem impossible to believe life exists in this barren place.

This illusion of death is necessary for life to flourish in a winter forest. The snow keeps the winter plants insulated and provides moisture for the harsh conditions. Frigid temperatures limit pests that would damage fragile plants and bacteria that cause disease. Trees and plants lie dormant and rest from growing. Like a deep sleep, this rest builds the plants' energy, enabling fresh growth and strengthening the plant to produce more seeds and fruit. **The lie of death hides the reality of life.**

Likewise, your shame is a lie with the appearance of death, making you believe you are incapable, unworthy, a failure, with no hope for success or life. It is a lie so loud, supported by so much false evidence, that you do not question it. Why would you seek another answer? If you are convinced a lie is truth, your thoughts and actions will defend the belief. Abundant life may seem impossible, but if you overcome the lie of your winter, you will find purpose and life.

Knowing God's truth **unravels lies** and **removes their power**. You must keep your mind stayed on His Word and the truth of who you are in Christ. **To overcome your labels, you must have different thoughts.** You must **choose** to consider yourself as God sees you.

When you perceive yourself as not____ enough (good enough, smart enough, thin enough, successful enough, etc.), remember God is not finished yet. **You are enough for God.** When you seem to fail, remember God makes you victorious. Mistakes do not equal failure. When you are unable, know it is God who makes you able. When you feel broken, remember that you are being healed. When you are scared, remember you are protected. **Surrender your old, broken self to the Lord and let Him redefine you!**

It is hard to love yourself
when you are deceived about who you are.

Take these five steps to stop the lies:

1. **Give up** your mess to God.

2. **Identify** the truth—the report of the Lord.

3. **Remind** yourself of that truth.

4. **Recognize** the report the enemy speaks to you.

5. **Stop** believing the lies!

<u>Questions to Ponder</u>

40.1) Who is good enough?

40.2) How have you let your mistakes define you? Do you trust that what the Lord says defines you? Why or why not?

40.3) In what ways do you recognize the Lord working in your heart to redefine some labels you have been believing?

40.4) How do you struggle to see the Lord working to change you? What is stopping that change?

40.5) What must you overcome to surrender to these changes?

40.6) List everything you like about yourself, especially regarding your character.

Open the lists you had others make about you in the homework from the last lesson.

40.7) What are the similarities to your lists?

40.8) Which of their answers are not on your list?

40.9) Do their answers surprise you? Why or why not?

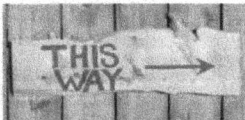

Ask your coach for more information about who you are in Christ

Visit the website at:

www.rebuiltrecovery.org

for downloadable pages and
more helpful resources!